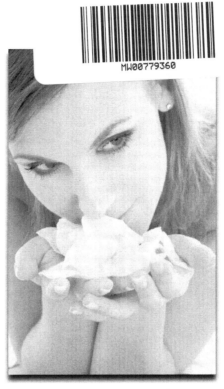

A DIY Guide to Therapeutic Spa Treatments

*Homemade Spa Recipes for
the Face, Hands, Feet and Body*
(The Art of the Bath Vol. 4)

Alynda Carroll

Ordinary Matters Publishing
P.O. Box 430577
Houston, TX 77243

www.OrdinaryMattersPublishing.com

A DIY Guide to Therapeutic Spa Treatments
Homemade Spa Recipes for the Face, Hands, Feet and Body

ISBN-13: 978-1-941303-11-5 (paperback)
ISBN-10: 1941303110
First Printing: October, 2014

Disclaimer and Terms of Use: Although the author and publisher have made every effort to ensure that the information in this book was correct at press time, the author and publisher to not assume and hereby disclaim any liability to any party for any loss, damage, or disruption caused by errors or omissions, whether such omissions result from negligence, accident, or any other cause. The author and the publisher do not warrant the accuracy of the information, text, and graphics contained within the book due to the rapidly changing nature of science, research, known and unknown facts, and the Internet. This book is presented solely for informational and entertainment purposes only.

Printed in the United States of America

Books by Alynda Carroll

The Art of the Bath Series

Custom Massage Therapy Oils
A DIY Guide to Therapeutic Recipes for Homemade Massage Oils

A DIY Guide to Therapeutic Bath Enhancements
Homemade Recipes for Bath Salts, Melts, Bombs & Scrubs

A DIY Guide to Therapeutic Body & Skin Care Recipes
Homemade Body Lotions, Skin Creams, Gels, Whipped Butters,
Herbal Balms and Salves

A DIY Guide to Therapeutic Spa Treatments
Homemade Recipes for the Face, Hands, Feet & Body

A DIY Guide to Therapeutic Body Butters
A Beginner's Guide to Homemade Body and Hair Butters

A DIY Guide to Therapeutic Natural Hair Care Recipes
A Beginner's Guide to Homemade Shampoos, Conditioners,
Rinses, Gels and Sprays

Life Hacks for Everyday Living Series

HOUSEHOLD HACKS
Super Simple Ways to Clean Your Home Effortlessly Using
Hydrogen Peroxide and Other Cleaning Secrets

Pick up your FREE report *Learn the Art of Self-Massage*:

http://www.ordinarymatterspublishing.com/massage-bonus

Praise for *The Art of the Bath* series

for *A DIY Guide to Therapeutic Spa Treatments from the Comfort of Your Home*

"*Ahhhh this is a keeper! It's packed with awesome and easy to make spa like treatments. I love going to the spa, but in between spa treatments this book is as good as it gets. My favorites so far are the healthy coconut cuticle softener, the tension-relieving eucalyptus food massage oil treatment- so good oh and for a coffee junkie like me, the all-over coffee body scrub priceless! Great DIY spa treatments book.*"
 ~ Yvette (Amazon reviewer)

for *A DIY Guide to Therapeutic Bath Enhancements*

". . . easy to follow and very simple too. If you are looking for a book that you can easily follow and make you feel like a pro in no time when it comes to making soaps, bath salts and scrubs, this is the book to have!"
~ LH Thompson (Amazon reviewer)

for *Custom Massage Therapy Oils*

As well as being relaxing, the benefits of massage can be physical as well as mental. This book is a great little guide to their therapeutic benefits, how to make your own massage oil and which blends are recommended to induce sleep, invigorate or enliven, boost the immune system and more. I will be taking the advice in this book on board, as I know how wonderful massage oils can be - it's just a case of knowing which ones are right to use, depending on the mood and/ or benefits you want to induce in the person receiving the massage." ~ Anna J (Amazon reviewer)

for *The Art of the Bath series*

"*I love Carroll's DIY Bath series. They are all so welcoming and are full of all these great ideas. Must have.*" ~ Laura Pope (Amazon reviewer)

"We delight in the beauty of a butterfly, but rarely admit the changes it has gone through to achieve that beauty."

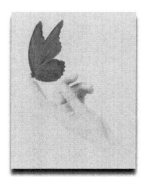

~ Maya Angelou

A Note to the Reader

Have you ever gone to a spa? If you haven't, it's a wonderful experience. I hope you have the chance to go sometime soon, but let's face it: spa-going is an expensive hobby.

I was lucky. My mom, like many women throughout history, made her own natural beauty recipes. She watched her mom use tried-and-true kitchen ingredients to take care of her own face, neck, and skin. My grandmother always wore a hat when she ventured out to avoid the sun and always made sure she included her neck when she moisturized her face. My mother would often talk about that famous scene in the movie Funny Girl, where Barbara Streisand grabbed lemon halves and rubbed them on her knees and elbows to lighten them. Baskets of lemons held a place of honor in our kitchen.

Neither my mother nor my grandmother ever went to a real spa, but they managed to create a pretty good replica of one at home. Homemade beauty recipes are a tradition in my family. It shouldn't be too surprising to learn that I'm a devotee, too.

Spending time luxuriating at a spa may seem like a dream you'll never be able to afford, but with a few inexpensive ingredients that you may already have, you can enjoy a spa day whenever you want.

Many of you may be familiar with my earlier books in the Art of the Bath series where I shared recipes for custom blended massage oils, bath enhancements like bombs, melts, salts, and scrubs, and homemade recipes for lotions, creams, whipped butters, and herbals and salves. I thought now would be a great time to take a look at the whole spa experience.

The recipes included in this book will allow you to give yourself treatments similar to those at exclusive spas, but do them in your own home. You don't have to wait until you have enough money in the bank to check in to the nearest professional spa or travel across states and continents. Create your own. Have the spa experience you've always dreamed of right now.

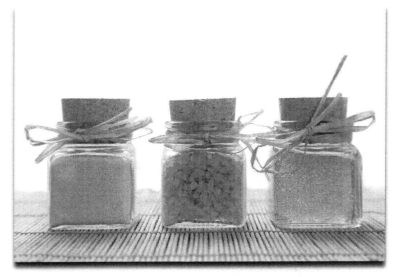

How to Give Yourself a Massage

Thank you for buying this book. In appreciation, I'm offering you this free report:

Learn the Art of Self-Massage

http://www.ordinarymatterspublishing.com/massage-bonus/

CONTENTS

INTRODUCTION

"The art of resting the mind and the power of dismissing from it all care and worry is probably one of the secrets of energy in our great men."

—Capt. J.A. Hadfield

What began as visits to mineral springs for their healing powers as far back as prehistoric times has turned into a spa industry that includes luxurious personal retreats and day-long personal care treatments. In addition to mediation practices, special foods and fitness regimens, today's spa experience isn't complete without facials, massages, and baths to beautify the face, hands, feet, and body. Treatments include those which exfoliate, detoxify, moisturize, and tone the skin and body. The recipes in this book are great way for you to have your own personal spa days.

There are also many therapeutic benefits to using the spa treatments in this book. These include relaxing tense muscles, relieving stress, increasing circulation, and strengthening the immune system.

Besides the beautifying and therapeutic benefits of spa treatments, these therapies can also be as much a balm to the spirit as it is to the body. Everyone deserves to take some personal time, to unwind and release the burdens of work and responsibilities. By using these treatments, you'll feel pampered and peaceful.

The Main Ingredients

With a few products that you may already have or that can be purchased at your local grocery or drug store, you can give yourself many of the same treatments you would receive at a high-end day spa. The main ingredients you will need include:

Salts – Epsom salts and sea salts contain beneficial minerals that aid in reducing inflammation and releasing toxins that build up in the body.

Oils – Mineral- and plant-based oils contain emollient qualities to smooth and moisturize dry or irritated skin.

Distilled Water – This is water that has had all chemicals or elements that could irritate the skin.

Clays – Clays are good for drawing out dirt beneath the skin and removing dead skin cells to leave skin feeling smoother and softer.

Essential oils – These plant-derived oils are potent and add the element of aromatherapy to treatments. They should be used with caution, especially if you are pregnant. Essential oils should not be used for products for children.

SAFETY FIRST!

Always use sterile utensils when creating products that will come in contact with the skin, especially if you have very sensitive skin.

Most treatments are designed to be used on every part of the body, but there are a few in this book that should not be used on the face.

It is important to try a small amount on the skin to see if there is a reaction before using on a larger area. This is especially true when using essential oils.

Women who are pregnant should double-check the warnings and side effects for all essential oils. Some oils should not be used during pregnancy.

If you take those few things into consideration as you move forward, I'm sure you'll agree that spa treatments are fun, easy to make, and will have you feel pampered in no time

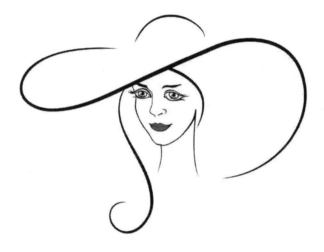

Treatments for the Face

RELAXING EUCALYPTUS FACIAL WRAP

After cleansing, a hot facial wrap can open pores to allow toxins and dirt under the surface of the skin escape. Eucalyptus oil is known to have beneficial effects as a muscle relaxant. How many of us feel those tensed facial muscles at the end of a long day? This is a great recipe to calm the mind and relax the body.

Ingredients:
2 cups distilled water
10 drops Eucalyptus essential oil
Soft dish cloth or large wash cloth

Directions:

Pour 2 cups of distilled water into a pan or bowl. Heat water on top of the stove or in a microwave until hot (not hot enough to burn, but hot to the touch). Add eucalyptus essential oil until desired scent strength is achieved. Place wash cloth in the water until completely saturated. Wring out excess water, leaving the cloth damp, but not dripping.

Drape on the face, leaving mouth and nostrils exposed. Leave on for 5 minutes. Pat dry.

EXFOLIATING FRENCH CLAY MASK

French clay is the main ingredient of that green mask you always see in photos, along with those sliced cucumbers over the eyes. It's all about green. Minerals in the clay account for French clay's distinctive color. This is a great mask to use after you have steamed your face and opened all the pores. Now, it's time to apply the mask so that the pores are tightened and the skin is toned. You'll find the gentle abrasiveness of the clay's fine granules make it an effective way to exfoliate as well. Great for all skin types, too.

Ingredients:
1/4 cup French Clay
2 tbsp Distilled water
10 drops Spearmint essential oil
Soft wash cloth
Warm water

Directions:

Place the French clay in a small bowl or cup. Stir in water a little at a time until a paste is formed. Add essential oil until desired scent strength is achieved. Consistency should be like that of pudding, so add more or less water until this is reached.

Apply to clean, dry face. Cover all parts of the face except the thin skin directly under eyes. Leave on 10 minutes or until mask is completely dry and tight.

Dampen the washcloth with warm water and lay over the face until mask is loosened a bit. Wipe mask off with horizontal strokes on the forehead and upward strokes from the chin to the brow. Gentle wiping is best.

When the entire mask has been removed, rinse the face in warm water and pat dry.

SOOTHING CUCUMBER MASK

I'm a huge fan of cucumbers when it comes to facial ingredients. Cucumbers are wonderful for the skin and especially for the face. The high amount of antioxidants and silica help in rejuvenating the skin and improving your complexion. You'll love the way this mask smoothes and softens the skin, too. The addition of full fat yogurt in the mask adds to the effect and helps all those tiny tense facial muscles relax. This is a great mask to use after spending a day out in the hot summer sun. If you're feeling playful, why not mash up about five leaves of fresh mint and add them to the mixture. The cucumber mask is another one that is good for all skin types.

Ingredients:
1/2 Cucumber, peeled
1 1/2 tbsp Plain full-fat yogurt

Directions:

In a food processer or blender, place cucumber and yogurt and puree until smooth.

Apply the mixture evenly over a smooth, dry face. Leave on for 15 minutes.

To remove, gently wipe off with a soft, dry wash cloth. After removing completely, rinse face in tepid water and pat dry.

CLEANSING LEMON FACIAL MASK

Do you have oily skin? You'll love this mask. The citric acid in lemons acts as an astringent in this mask, while the Fuller's Earth Clay is highly absorbent, making it especially beneficial to anyone who has oily skin. The lemon mask is also a great cleansing mask for any skin type.

Ingredients:
1/4 cup Fuller's Earth Clay
2 tbsp Freshly squeezed lemon juice
2 tbsp Distilled water
Soft wash cloth
Warm water

Directions:

In a small bowl or cup, stir together all of the ingredients, adding as much water as it takes to create a pudding-like texture.

Apply the mixture to a clean, dry face. Smooth on the face evenly, being careful not to put on the thin skin under the eyes. Leave on for 10 minutes or until the mask dries and tightens.

To remove, dampen a wash cloth in warm water and place over face for a few minutes or until mask becomes loose. Gently wipe the mask off using horizontal stokes on the forehead and upward strokes from the chin to the brow line.

After all the mask is removed, rinse face with clean, warm water. Pat dry.

REPLENISHING AVOCADO FACE MASK

Today avocados are highly touted for all their many health benefits. Full of the rich vitamins A, D, and E as well as oils that are similar to those found in the skin, avocados are equally enriching for the face. Avocado masks are beneficial for all skin types because of the way they moisturize skin, but anyone with dry skin will love how this mask helps to heal, soothe, and replenish their dry skin.

Ingredients:
1 Ripe avocado
2 tsp Full-fat plain yogurt
1 tsp Honey
Soft wash cloth

Directions:

Mash avocado in a small bowl. While stirring, add in yogurt and honey, until a smooth paste is formed.

Apply the mixture to a clean, dry face. Leave on for 10 minutes.

To remove, wipe off with soft wash cloth. After all the mask is removed, rinse face with warm water and pat dry.

Treatments for the Hands

HEALTHY COCONUT CUTICLE SOFTENER

To encourage healthy nail growth, cuticles should be pushed back regularly. As well as making it easier to do this, Vitamin E oil is wonderful and a great oil to have on hand. For good nail health, use this homemade cuticle softener. The Vitamin E oil will help to soothe and heal dry cracking skin that surrounds the nail.

Ingredients:
1 tsp Vitamin E oil
1 tsp Coconut oil
Q-tips
Soft, dry wash cloth

Directions:

Mix oils together in a small bowl or cup. Using a Q-tip, dab oil on each cuticle and around the nail bed. Gently, massage each nail, to work oil into cuticle. Using a soft wash cloth, gently push back each cuticle. Once all cuticles have been pushed back, use any remaining oil to massage each finger or any dry areas. Wipe hands off with cloth and then wash with soap and water to remove excess oil.

SIMPLE and CREAMY MILK HAND SOAK

I'm sure you've heard of the many benefits milk brings to skin care, but have you thought about using it for nail care? Milk contains lactic acid that can be very beneficial to the skin, including moisturizing the skin, removing dead cells, and soothing dried or cracked skin. As an alternative, try buttermilk to strengthen those nails. You can also add a little salt for an added exfoliation factor.

Ingredients:
1 cup Whole milk
1 cup Heavy whipping cream

Directions:

In a bowl large enough to place both hands, mix milk and cream. Heat in the microwave until warm (not hot). Place hands in the milk and soak for 5 minutes.

BROWN SUGAR and ALMOND HAND SCRUB

This recipe uses another handy kitchen ingredient, brown sugar. Sugar is good for the skin due to its light abrasive action. Couple the use of this scrub with a good hand soak and you'll find your hands feeling even more soft and smooth. With brown sugar, you get the addition of molasses which makes this sugar scrub less abrasive but just as effective as other types of scrubs. For a twist, switch to coconut or olive,

Ingredients:
2/3 cup Brown sugar
1/3 cup Almond oil

Directions:

In a bowl, place brown sugar. Add oil, combining as you go, until the mixture is the consistency of damp sand.

Gather a handful of the mixture and rub all over your hands. Be sure and pay extra attention to any dry patches. Rinse hands with warm water.

19

LEMON LIGHT HAND SCRUB

Nothing beats the fresh scent of lemons. One of the major benefits for the skin is the slight bleaching quality offered by the lemon. Lemons have been used for generations to lighten brown spots found on the hands. You'll find your hands smoother and revitalized after a good lemon scrub. You might just be in a better mood, too.

Ingredients:
2/3 cup White granulated sugar
1/3 cup Olive oil
2 tbsp Freshly squeezed lemon juice

Directions:

In a bowl, place sugar. While stirring, add mineral oil until mixture is the consistency of damp sand. Stir in lemon juice.

Gather a handful and rub onto hands until they are completely covered. Gently rub on any rough patches. Rinse hands with warm water afterwards.

COCONUT HAND TREATMENT

Coconut oil is praised for its many benefits. I think the oil must be one of the biggest multitaskers around. Everywhere you look someone is alluding to yet another new reason to give this oil a try. So, I imagine it's become a staple in today's kitchen. When it comes to skin, coconut oil is rich in fats and emollients that can heal even the driest hands. If you want smooth, supple skin, use coconut oil. Don't make the mistake of thinking more is better. The skin will only absorb so much and the rest will just rest on top. Agave nectar is known for its anti-bacterial properties. Many promote its use for anti-aging. Combine the two and you have a quick but powerful treatment for the hands.

Ingredients:
1/2 cup Coconut oil
1 tbsp Agave nectar
Cotton gloves

Directions:

Mix the coconut oil and agave nectar in a bowl until completely combined. Gather some of the mixture and rub all over hands. Put on cotton gloves. Leave gloves on for 30 minutes. Remove gloves and rinse hands in warm water.

Treatments for the Feet

TRIED and TRUE SOOTHING FOOT SOAK

Sometimes all you really need is a simple, well-documented remedy that works. No muss, no fuss. That's what you get when you combine Epsom salts with water. Yes, everyone knows this one, but pretty much everyone forgets. The next time you're feeling that aching fatigue after a long day of work, grab a pan, some water, and some Epsom salts. Nothing feels better than a warm foot soak that relaxes the muscles in those tired feet. An added benefit is that Epsom salts contain magnesium sulfate, which can reduce inflammation and flush toxins from the body.

Ingredients:
1/2 cup Epsom salt
6 cups Warm water

Directions:

In a basin large enough to place your feet, pour in warm water. Stir in Epsom salts until dissolved. Place the feet in the basin and soak for 10 minutes. Remove and pat dry.

OLD-TIME VINEGAR FOOT SOAK

Apple cider vinegar has been used for centuries to reduce the spread of toenail fungus and in some cases get rid of it completely. The reason why is that apple cider vinegar contains acetic acid, which has been known to erode the enamel on teeth. This harsh quality is what makes it a beneficial exfoliator and defense against bacteria.

Ingredients:
2 cups Apple Cider vinegar
2 cups Warm Water
Pumice stone
Soft towel

Directions:

In a basin large enough to place feet, mix together vinegar and water. Soak feet for 30 minutes. Dry feet with soft towel and gently use pumice stone to remove calluses or rough patches. Place feet back in vinegar solution and soak for 5 more minutes. Remove and dry feet thoroughly.

LAVENDER and GINGER ULTRA SMOOTH FOOT TREATMENT

How are your feet doing? Is the skin getting tougher, even thicker? Here's a pretty good three-step treatment that should soften those tootsies of yours. A little preparation is needed for this one. You'll also have to figure out the best time of day to do this. Instead of the distilled water, you might want to try apple cider or apple cider vinegar. Lavender oil is known for its calming effect.

Ingredients:
2 tbsp Beeswax, grated
3 - 4 drops lavender essential oil
1/4 cup Distilled water
2 tbsp ginger, ground
2 cups White vinegar
2 gal hot water
Plastic bags large enough to cover each foot
Socks

Directions:

Step One: The Cream

Prepare the foot cream ahead of time: Mix together the lavender oil and the beeswax. Heat slowly in a double boiler until the mixture has melted but has not reached the boiling point.

In a microwave-safe container, heat the distilled water for about one minute, right before it boils. Slowly mix the heated water to the mixture. Add the ginger.

Step Two: The Soak

Combine vinegar and heated water. Soak feet for about 45 minutes. Rub feet dry to remove any dry skin or calluses.

Step Three:

Slather both feet with the prepared Lavender and Ginger foot cream. Make sure all the skin is covered. Then place each foot in a plastic bag and then slip the socks over the bags. Wear the sock-covered treatment for a few hours before cleaning feet. Feet should be ultra-smooth. .

HONEY FOOT SCRUB

Honey is another one of those ingredients with a huge pedigree. Honey is a great addition to any scrub. The rice granules glide evenly over the foot and produce a gentle way to exfoliate the feet. You'll have to do a little work to create the scrub, but it's worth it.

Ingredients:
1 cup Rice
2 tbsp Honey
1 tbsp Olive oil

Directions:

Place rice in food processor and blend until it becomes flour-like. In a bowl, mix the rice flour with the honey and oil to a paste consistency.

Rub the paste all over feet, massaging into the soles and heels well. Rinse with warm water to remove.

TENSION-RELIEVING EUCALYPTUS FOOT MASSAGE OIL

On a daily basis, the arch muscles of the foot take the most abuse of any other muscle in the body. Massaging this area of the foot can lessen tension and relieve these sore aching muscles.

Ingredients:
4 tsp Jojoba oil
6 drops Eucalyptus essential oil

Directions:

For every 4 teaspoons of Jojoba oil, add 6 drops of Eucalyptus oil until there is enough to rub on both feet. Apply generously and rub with gentle pressure into the feet, concentrating on the arch, ball, and heel of the foot. Towel off feet when finished.

Store left over oil in a dark container.

Treatments for the Body

CLASSIC DETOX BATH

Salt baths are very beneficial to the skin including relaxing tight muscles, reducing inflammation and flushing out toxins. If possible, use Dead Sea salts, which are extremely dense in mineral content. You'll enjoy taking a detox bath and cleansing the body of all its toxins. Be sure you follow the suggestions to start slowly and increase the soaking time incrementally so that your body gets accustomed to the process. .

Ingredients:
1 cup Sea Salt
1 cup Epsom Salt

Directions:

In a warm bath, mix salts until dissolved. Soak in the bath for 10 minutes. Increase the amount of time you soak by 5 minutes each time you bathe until you are soaking for 30 minutes.

ROYAL ROSE-SCENTED MILK BATH

When it comes to major pampering, a milk bath is one of those timeless remedies for a luxurious, relaxing bath. This is the bath of the royals. None other than the great Queen Cleopatra has sung the praises of the milk bath. In addition to being the ultimate relaxation therapy, a milk bath will soften the entire body.

Ingredients:
2 1/2 cups Whole powdered milk
1/2 Cornstarch
12 drops Rose essential oil
1/4 cup Dried rose petals (optional)

Directions:

In a bowl, mix together powdered milk and cornstarch. Stir in, drop by drop, the rose essential oil, until desired scent strength is achieved. Pour mixture under running water into bath. Sprinkle in rose petals. Soak for as long as you like.

ALL-OVER COFFEE BODY SCRUB

If you're a coffee junkie like me, this scrub is going to receive a lot of attention, but don't worry if you aren't. Coffee has a good many attributes and is a perfect addition to a beauty recipe. Fine ground coffee makes a great exfoliator and is known to rejuvenate the skin by increasing circulation. You'll have to play around to get the right amount that you'll need.

Ingredients:
3/4 cup Coffee (finely ground)
1/4 cup Granulated sugar
1/4 cup Olive oil

Directions:

For every 3/4 cup of coffee grounds, add 1/4 cup sugar and 1/4 cup of oil, combining together to form a paste. Smooth over the body, and rubbing in circular motions, especially on the heels, knees, elbows and shoulders. Rinse with water that is warm to remove.

SIMPLE LAVENDER SUGAR BODY SCRUB

Lavender oil is such a great ingredient when you want to add a dash of relaxation to any recipe. Keep in mind that raw sugar is an extremely coarse exfoliator and should not be used on the face -- body only.

Ingredients:
2 cups Raw sugar
1/2 cup White refined sugar
1 tbsp Honey
1/2 cup Extra virgin olive oil
10 drops Lavender essential oil

Directions:

In a medium bowl, mix the sugars together. Stir in honey and olive oil. Add, drop by drop, lavender essential oil until desired scent strength is reached. Apply to the body and rub in a circular motion to exfoliate. Rinse to remove.

AFTER-THE-BATH OVERALL BODY OIL

This is a great oil to use after a bath or shower when all the pores are open. Use this oil when you want to rehydrate and moisturize your body. Make sure you apply this oil while the skin is still wet. You'll love taking in the relaxing aroma of lavender as you smooth the oil all over.

Ingredients:
1/2 cup Olive oil
12 drops Lavender essential oil

Directions:

In a plastic cup or container, mix together mineral oil and essential oil. While skin is still wet, apply generously on the body, rubbing in well. Towel dry

Conclusion

We've come to the end of our journey. What could be better than a personal retreat at a luxurious spa? Creating your own at-home spa day! I hope you've been inspired enough to start planning yours. As you can tell by the list of ingredients, this will be way less-expensive than a trip to the neighborhood day spa or a fancy hotel spa.

As you've seen, it takes very little to replicate some of the most expensive treatments provided within the walls of the most lavish spas in the world. You'll find most of the ingredients right in your own pantry. Why not plan to take an entire day just or you, a day to eat healthier, drink better, and immerse yourself in the world of a spa by pampering yourself with some of the treatments in this book. After all, don't you deserve a little "me" time?

Thank you for taking the time to read through these recipes. Be sure and look for my other books that arc part of the "art of the bath" series. I also hope you've enjoyed the book enough to share it with others. If you did, please a leave an honest positive review on the book's sales page.

Be sure and look for my other books that relate to the whole "art of the bath" experience and tell others.

Alynda Carroll

P.S: I hope you've enjoyed this book and will take a few minutes to leave a review. Reviews are a big help for authors as well as readers.

About the Author

Alynda Carroll has loved baths since she was a little
Bubble baths, lotions, and creams have fascinated her.
spent many hours watching her mom create homema
beauty recipes. Later, Alynda's interests expanded to incluc
herbs, essential oils, aromatherapy and the art of the bath as i
is today.

Be sure and buy the rest of Alynda Carroll's best-selling
books that make up her popular series The Art of the Bath, s
well as her new series Life Hacks for Everyday Living. Look
for the excerpt from her new book HOUSEHOLD HACKS
at the back of this book.

girl.
She
de
e

MORE BOOKS BY ALYNDA CARROLL

The Art of the Bath Series

Custom Massage Therapy Oils: A DIY Guide to Therapeutic Recipes for Homemade Massage Oils

A DIY Guide to Therapeutic Bath Enhancements: Homemade Recipes for Bath Salts, Melts, Bombs & Scrubs

A DIY Guide to Therapeutic Body & Skin Care Recipes: Homemade Body Lotions, Skin Creams, Gels, Whipped Butters, Herbal Balms & Salves

A DIY Guide to Therapeutic Spa Treatments: Homemade Recipes for the Face, Hands, Feet & Body

A DIY Guide to Therapeutic Body Butters: A Beginner's Guide to Homemade Body and Hair Butters

A DIY Guide to Therapeutic Natural Hair Care Recipes: A Beginner's Guide to Homemade Shampoos, Conditioners, Rinses, Gels and Sprays

Life Hacks for Everyday Living *(New Series)*

HOUSEHOLD HACKS: Super Simple Ways to Clean Your Home Effortlessly Using Hydrogen Peroxide and Other Cleaning Secrets

What's New?

Turn the page to read an excerpt from HOUSEHOLD HACKS. To receive updates on the release of Alynda Carroll's next books in the Art of the Bath series and BEAUTY HACKS, go to:

www.SimpleLivingHacks.com

Excerpt from
HOUSEHOLD HACKS

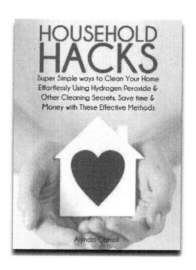

Welcome to Household Hacks, my personal collection of more than 200 cleaning tips, tricks, and household hacks for all areas of the home with an emphasis on using natural, inexpensive cleaners and strategies. Many have been around for a long time, but others are focused on the way we live today.

The advantages are many. You'll save money, time, and energy. You'll also become more effective at housecleaning by using these tips and strategies that will free up your time.

You'll find information about well-seasoned natural cleaners that have been helping people clean for generations and understand why they are gaining popularity today.

You'll discover cleaning strategies and hacks for various rooms including the kitchen, bathroom, and bedroom, as well as the home office. You'll even find creative living hacks to make home life easier.

This collection captures my favorites and includes additional hints and alternatives. If you already have a deep interest in DIY household hacks and natural cleaners, you will probably come across some familiar cleaning remedies. They will serve as reminders, but be of more interest to readers who are just starting down this more natural and simplified way of living. However, newer strategies and ideas will encourage you on your own journey toward living a more natural, clean, and simple life.

A major plus about having this book is that everything is gathered in this one place. This is a good, fun, and definitely useful reference to have on hand.

How the Book is Organized

The book begins by taking a look at the top natural cleaners in use today. There are several cleaning hacks and tips for each cleaner. I like to have a list of things I can do with a particular cleaner, as well as a collection of cleaning tips particular to an area of the home. The second section offers additional cleaning suggestions and creative household hacks for the kitchen, bathroom, bedroom, laundry and closet, living room, home office, and, by extension, the car.

❑ Natural Cleaners
❑ Hydrogen Peroxide
❑ Vinegar
❑ Baking Soda
❑ Lemon and lemon juice
❑ Apple Cider Vinegar
❑ Salt
❑ Household Hacks
❑ Office and Technology
❑ Bathroom
❑ Kitchen
❑ Bedroom
❑ Laundry and Closet
❑ Car
❑ Creative Hacks

Now that you have an idea of what *HOUSEHOLD HACKS* contains, are you ready to discover its treasures?

Buy your copy of *HOUSEHOLD HACKS* today.
www.SimpleLivingHacks.com

NOTES

INDEX

Made in the USA
San Bernardino, CA
22 March 2015